RISE AGAIN

The Road to Recovery for Painful Joints

Mills K. Owen

TABLE OF CONTENT

Introduction

Tom was a former athlete who loved to play basketball and run marathons. However, as he got older, his joints started to ache and he found it increasingly difficult to stay active. He had tried various pain medications, physical therapy, and other treatments, but nothing seemed to bring him lasting relief.

One day, I recommended my strategies in this book "Rise Again: The Road to Recovery for Painful Joints." Tom was skeptical at first but decided to give it a try. As he read through this book, he was fascinated by the information on the causes of joint pain and the various remedies that were available. He was especially intrigued by the mind-body techniques and the role that exercise and physical therapy could play in managing his pain.

Tom decided to take the advice in this book and make some changes to his lifestyle. He started by incorporating daily stretches and exercises into his routine and focusing on eating a healthy, anti-inflammatory diet. He also started practicing mindfulness and meditation to reduce stress and improve his overall well-being.

Within a few weeks, Tom began to notice a difference. His pain was less intense and he was able to move more easily. He continued to follow the principles in this book and gradually increased his activity level. Before long, he was able to play basketball and run marathons again, just like he used to.

Tom was amazed by the impact that this book had on his life. He felt like a new man and was grateful to have found a solution to his joint pain. He recommended this book to all of his friends who were struggling with joint pain, and many of them had similar experiences of relief and recovery.

In the end, Tom was grateful for the guidance and inspiration he had found in "Rise Again: The Road to Recovery for Painful Joints." He knew that he would continue to use the techniques and principles from the book to keep his joints healthy and strong for years to come.

Joint pain can be a debilitating and life-altering experience. Whether you suffer from a recent injury, an underlying medical condition, or simply the wear and tear of aging, joint pain can limit your mobility, impact your quality of life, and leave you feeling frustrated and helpless.

However, there is hope. With the right approach, it is possible to manage joint pain, rebuild your body, and reclaim your life. In this book, you will learn about the causes of joint pain, the anatomy of joints, and the various medical and natural remedies that are available for pain management.

You will also discover how to use exercise, physical therapy, and mind-body techniques to rebuild your strength and prevent future injury. Whether you are a seasoned athlete, an older adult, or anyone in between, this book will provide you with the tools and guidance you need to rise again and reclaim your life.

So let's start if you are prepared to get control over your joint discomfort. You will overcome joint discomfort and have a healthy, active, and meaningful life if you have the correct information and motivation.

Chapter 1

The Causes of Joint Pain

Common sources of joint pain can include:

1. **Arthritis:** Arthritis is a common cause of joint pain and is a term used to describe inflammation of the joint. The two most common types of arthritis are osteoarthritis and rheumatoid arthritis, both of which can cause pain, swelling, stiffness and loss of range of motion in the joints.

2. **Injury or Trauma:** Joints can be damaged by a single traumatic event,

such as a fall, or by repetitive stress, such as from overuse during sports activities. Joint pain can also be caused by muscle strains and sprains, ligament tears and joint dislocations.

3. **Infection:** Joints can also be affected by infection, most commonly in the form of septic arthritis. This is caused by bacteria, fungi or viruses entering the joint, leading to inflammation and pain.

4. **Overuse:** Overuse injuries can result from repetitive activities such as running, tennis or golf. This type of joint pain is often the result of a tendon or ligament being strained or

tendinitis, which is an inflammation of the tendon.

Factors that contribute to joint pain and injury include:

1. **Age:** Age is one of the most common factors associated with joint pain and injury. As people age, their joints begin to wear down and become less flexible, leading to increased stiffness and pain.

2. **Overuse:** Overuse injuries are common in athletes, particularly those involved in repetitive activities such as running, tennis, or golf. Repetitive motions can cause the tendons and ligaments to become inflamed, leading to pain and stiffness.

3. **Poor Posture:** Poor posture can lead to misalignment of the spine and joints, causing them to become strained and leading to pain and discomfort.

4. **Obesity:** Excess weight puts extra strain on the joints, leading to increased pain and stiffness.

5. **Lack of Exercise:** Regular exercise is important for keeping the joints flexible and strong. Without regular exercise, the joints become weaker and more prone to injury.

How to identify the root cause of your joint pain

Identifying the root cause of your joint pain can be a challenge, but it is essential to finding the right treatment plan. Here are some tips on how to identify the root cause of your joint pain:

1. **Keep a Pain Journal:** Keeping a pain journal can help you track any changes in your joint pain, such as what activities seem to make it worse or better, when it occurs, and how long it lasts. This can help you and your doctor narrow down the source of your pain.

2. **Talk to Your Doctor:** Your doctor can help you determine the cause of your joint pain. Be sure to discuss all of your symptoms, including any associated pain and stiffness.

3. **Consider Other Causes:** Joint pain can also be caused by other conditions such as infection, injury, or arthritis. If

you have any of these conditions, your doctor may suggest further testing.

4. **Get a Second Opinion**: If you're not sure what's causing your joint pain, you may want to consider getting a second opinion from a specialist. By taking the time to properly identify the root cause of your joint pain, you can develop a treatment plan that works for you and help you get back to living a pain-free life.

Understanding the structure and function of joints

Understanding the structure and function of joints is key to understanding joint pain and how to treat it. Joints are formed when two or more bones come together and are made up of tough connective tissue, cartilage, muscles, tendons, and ligaments. The purpose of joints is to provide movement, stability, and support for the body. The joint capsule is a tough, fibrous membrane that encases the joint, holding it together and providing protection from injury. Inside the joint capsule is a lubricating fluid known as synovial fluid, which helps reduce friction and provides nourishment to the cartilage.

Cartilage is a soft tissue found on the ends of bones that helps absorb shock and provides cushioning for the joint. Muscles, tendons, and ligaments are all responsible for providing stability and support to the joint. Muscles are responsible for moving, while tendons and ligaments provide support and stability. Having an understanding of the anatomy and function of joints can help with diagnosing and treating joint pain.

Knowing the structure and function of the joint can help determine the cause of the pain and the best treatment options.
Common types of joint injuries and their effects include:

1. **Sprains:** A sprain occurs when a ligament is stretched or torn, resulting in pain, swelling, and instability in the joint.

2. **Strains:** A strain occurs when a muscle or tendon is overstretched or torn, resulting in pain and difficulty moving the joint.

3. **Dislocations:** Dislocations occur when a bone is forced out of its joint, resulting in pain, swelling, instability, and inability to move the joint.

4. **Fractures:** Fractures occur when a bone is broken, resulting in pain, swelling, instability, and inability to move the joint.

5. **Tendinitis:** Tendinitis is an inflammation of a tendon, resulting in pain, swelling, and difficulty moving the joint.

How to assess the severity of a joint injury

Assessing the severity of a joint injury is important to determine the best course of treatment. The following are helpful tips for assessing the severity of a joint injury:

1. Check for pain, swelling, and discoloration of the affected joint.

2. Check for instability or inability to move the joint.

3. Check for any deformity of the joint.

4. Check for any associated symptoms, such as numbness or tingling.

5. Check for any signs of infection, such as redness or warmth in the area.

Chapter 2

Medical Treatments for Joint Pain

Overview of available medical treatments for painful joints:

The good news is that there are a variety of medical treatments available for people suffering from painful joints. From medications to physical therapy, orthopedic surgery to alternative treatments, there is something to help everyone find relief.

Medications come in a variety of forms, from over-the-counter pain relievers to prescription anti-inflammatory drugs.

Physical therapy can help strengthen the muscles around the joint, improving joint function and reducing pain.

Orthopedic surgery is an option for more severe cases, and alternative treatments such as acupuncture, massage, and herbal remedies have been known to help.

Pros and Cons of Common Treatments for Painful Joints:

Pain medications: Pros – Pain medications can offer fast relief from painful joints, and are available over the counter or with a prescription. Cons – Pain medications can be habit-forming and may cause side effects such as abdominal pain, diarrhea, and nausea.

Physical therapy: Pros – Physical therapy can help strengthen the muscles around the joint and improve joint function. Cons – Physical therapy can be expensive and time consuming.

Surgery: Pros – Surgery can be an effective treatment for more severe cases of painful joints. Cons – Surgery is expensive and carries risks such as infection and scarring.

How to work with your doctor to develop a treatment plan that is right for you:

If you are suffering from painful joints, it is important to consult with your doctor to develop a treatment plan that is right for you. Start by discussing your symptoms and medical history with your doctor. Make sure to tell your doctor about any medications you are taking, as well as any lifestyle changes you have made to try to relieve your pain.

Your doctor can then help you decide on the best course of treatment based on your individual needs. Together, you can work to develop a treatment plan that is tailored to your specific needs, and that will help you find relief from your painful joints.

Natural Remedies for Joint Pain

Some natural herbs that may help relieve joint pain include:

Turmeric: Contains curcumin, which has anti-inflammatory properties. It can either be taken as a supplement or mixed into meals.

Turmeric: You can add turmeric to your food or take it in supplement form. The recommended dose is usually 500-2,000 mg per day.

Ginger: Also has anti-inflammatory properties and can be taken as a supplement or added to food.

Ginger: Ginger can be added to food or taken in supplement form. The recommended dose is usually 1-2 grams per day.

Boswellia: Also known as Indian frankincense, it can help reduce inflammation and pain. As a supplement, it can be used without risk.

Boswellia: Boswellia is typically taken in supplement form. The recommended dose is usually 300-500 mg, three times per day.

Devil's claw: Contains harpagoside, which has anti-inflammatory properties. As a supplement, it can be used without risk.

Devil's claw: Devil's claw is typically taken in supplement form. The recommended dose is usually 1,500 mg per day.

Willow bark: Contains salicin, which is similar to aspirin and can help relieve pain. As a supplement, it can be used without risk.

Willow bark: Willow bark is typically taken in supplement form. The recommended dose is usually 240 mg, two to three times per day.

Other natural remedies for joint pain include:

Omega-3 fatty acids: Found in fish and fish oil supplements, they can help reduce inflammation.

Glucosamine and chondroitin: Supplements that may help improve joint function and reduce pain.

Massage therapy: Can aid with flexibility improvement and pain reduction.

Acupuncture: May help relieve pain and improve joint function.

It's important to follow the recommended dosages for these herbs and to talk to your doctor before starting any new supplements or remedies, especially if you are pregnant, nursing, or taking any medications. Your doctor can help you determine the best course of action based on your individual needs and health status.

Chapter 3

Rebuilding Your Body: Exercise and Physical Therapy

Exercise is crucial for maintaining joint health for several reasons:

- **Improves Flexibility and Range of Motion:** Regular exercise can help improve the range of motion and flexibility of your joints, which can reduce the risk of injury and pain. Stretching and low-impact exercises, such as yoga and Pilates, are great options for increasing flexibility.

- **Strengthens Supporting Muscles:** Strong muscles around your joints can help support them and reduce stress on the joints. Resistance training and weightlifting can help improve muscle strength, which can in turn improve joint health.

- **Maintains Joint Strength:** Regular exercise can help maintain the strength of the bones, tendons, and ligaments that make up your joints. This is particularly important for people with conditions such as osteoporosis, which can cause bones to weaken.

- **Reduces Inflammation:** Exercise has been shown to reduce inflammation in the body, which can help reduce pain and improve joint health. Low-impact exercises, such as swimming and cycling, can be particularly helpful in reducing joint inflammation.

- **Improves Cartilage Health:** Cartilage is the cushioning material that helps reduce friction in your joints. Exercise can help improve the health of this cartilage, reducing the risk of joint damage and osteoarthritis.

In summary, exercise is an essential component of joint health, as it can help improve flexibility, strengthen supporting muscles, maintain joint strength, reduce inflammation, and improve cartilage health. It's important to consult with a doctor before starting a new exercise program, particularly if you have a pre-existing joint condition.

Physical therapy is an effective way to strengthen injured joints and prevent future injury. Here are some steps to follow:

Consult with a Physical Therapist: A physical therapist can help assess the injury and develop a treatment plan that is specific to your needs and goals. They will also guide proper form and technique during exercises to help prevent further injury.

Focus on Strengthening and Stabilizing Exercises: Physical therapy often involves a combination of exercises to strengthen the muscles and stabilize the joint. This can include resistance training, weightlifting, and bodyweight exercises. Your physical therapist can help you determine the appropriate level of resistance for your condition.

Incorporate Range of Motion Exercises: In addition to strengthening exercises, physical therapy may also include a range of motion exercises to improve flexibility and mobility. This can help reduce stiffness and prevent future injury.

Incorporate Balance and Proprioception Training: Physical therapists may also incorporate balance and proprioception training into their therapy. These exercises help improve your body's ability to sense and respond to changes in your environment, reducing the risk of falls and other injuries.

Gradually Increase Intensity: Physical therapy should be gradual, with the intensity of exercises increasing over time as your joint strength and stability improve. Your physical therapist can help you determine when it is appropriate to progress to more challenging exercises.

Use Assistive Devices: If necessary, your physical therapist may recommend using assistive devices, such as braces or crutches, to help protect the joint and support your progress during therapy.

Physical therapy is a valuable tool for strengthening injured joints and preventing future injury. Working with a physical therapist can help you safely and effectively regain strength and stability in your joints.

Here is a list of sample exercises and stretches that can target common problem areas:

Lower Back:

- **Cat-Cow Stretch:** Start on your hands and knees and alternate between arching your back and rounding it.

- **Knee-to-Chest Stretch:** Lie on your back and bring one knee toward your chest, holding for 20-30 seconds before repeating on the other side.

- **Superman Exercise:** Lie face down on the floor and lift your arms, legs, and chest off the ground.

Shoulders:

- **Shoulder Blade Squeeze:** Stand or sit with your shoulders back and down and squeeze your shoulder blades together.

- **Overhead Reach:** Stand with your arms overhead and reach up as high as you can, stretching the shoulders.

- **Doorway Stretch:** Stand in a doorway with your arms outstretched and lean forward, stretching the chest and shoulders.

Hips:

- **Figure Four Stretch:** Lie on your back and cross one ankle over the opposite knee, pulling the knee towards your chest.

- **Butterfly Stretch:** Sit with the soles of your feet together and gently press your knees toward the floor.

- **Lizard Pose:** Start in a high plank position and bring one knee to the outside of the same elbow.

Knees:

- **Hamstring Stretch:** Sit on the floor with one leg extended and reach forward to touch your toes.

- **Calf Stretch:** Stand facing a wall and place one foot behind the other, pressing your heel to the ground.

- **Quad Stretch:** Stand with one hand on a wall for balance and bend the knee to bring your heel towards your buttock.

Ankles:

- **Calf Raise:** Stand with your feet shoulder-width apart and raise onto the balls of your feet.

- **Ankle Circles:** Sit in a chair and rotate your ankle in a circular motion in both directions.

- **Ankle Pumps:** Lie on your back and move your ankle up and down, then side to side.

These exercises and stretches can help improve flexibility, reduce pain, and prevent injury in common problem areas. It's important to listen to your body and only do what you feel comfortable with and to consult with a doctor or physical therapist before starting any new exercise program.

Chapter 4

Mind-Body Approaches to Joint Pain

The connection between stress and joint pain

There is a complex relationship between stress and joint pain. Stress can cause physical tension in the body, which can lead to muscle tightness, inflammation, and joint pain. This is because stress activates the body's "fight or flight" response, which releases stress hormones such as cortisol and adrenaline that can increase inflammation and muscle tension.

Additionally, stress can also lead to changes in posture and behavior, such as clenching your jaw, grinding your teeth, or hunching over a computer, which can put additional strain on joints and cause pain.

On the other hand, joint pain can also cause stress. When you experience joint pain, it can affect your ability to perform everyday activities and cause discomfort, leading to feelings of anxiety and depression. There might be a complicated and inverse link between stress and joint discomfort.

Exercise, mindfulness practices, and relaxation methods may all be used to manage stress and lessen its negative effects on joint pain.

It's important to see a healthcare professional if you are dealing with joint pain and stress to create an effective treatment strategy.

Mindfulness and other mind-body techniques can be effective in managing pain and promoting healing by reducing stress and improving overall well-being.

Here are some techniques you can use:

- **Mindfulness Meditation:** Practicing mindfulness meditation involves focusing on the present moment and paying attention to your thoughts, feelings, and sensations without judgment. This can help reduce stress and anxiety and increase self-awareness, which can help you better understand and manage your pain.

- **Progressive Muscle Relaxation:** This method includes tensing and then relaxing each muscle group in your body, beginning at the bottom and working your way up to the top. This can help reduce muscle tension and reduce pain.

- **Deep Breathing:** Deep breathing can help calm the body and reduce stress and pain. You can practice deep breathing by taking slow, deep breaths, focusing on the sensation of the air moving in and out of your body.

- **Guided Imagery:** Guided imagery involves using your imagination to create a mental image of a peaceful, healing environment. This can help you relax and reduce pain by distracting you from the sensations of pain and allowing you to focus on something positive.

- **Yoga:** Yoga combines physical postures, breathing exercises, and mindfulness to improve physical and mental well-being. Gentle yoga poses can help increase flexibility, reduce stress, and improve joint health.

It's important to remember that these techniques may not work for everyone, and it's important to find what works best for you. It's also important to talk to your doctor before starting any new exercise program, especially if you have a chronic condition or are in pain. With time and practice, these techniques can be powerful tools in helping manage pain and promote healing.

Guidelines for lowering stress and enhancing general well-being

Reducing stress and improving overall well-being are important for managing pain and promoting healing. Here are some advice that you might find useful:

- **Exercise regularly:** Regular exercise can help reduce stress and improve overall well-being by releasing endorphins, the body's natural painkillers. Aim for 30 minutes of moderate physical activity, such as brisk walking, every day.

- **Get enough sleep:** A good night's sleep is important for reducing stress and improving overall well-being. Aim for 7-9 hours of sleep each night, and establish a regular sleep routine to help you fall asleep and stay asleep.

- **Eat a healthy diet:** A balanced diet rich in fruits, vegetables, whole grains, and lean protein can help improve overall well-being and reduce stress. Avoid processed and high-fat foods, and limit caffeine and alcohol.

- **Practice mindfulness:** Mindfulness techniques, such as meditation and deep breathing, can help reduce stress and improve overall well-being by calming the mind and reducing anxiety.

- **Connect with others:** Spending time with family and friends, volunteering, or joining a support group can help improve overall well-being by reducing stress and providing social support.

- **Manage time effectively:** Being able to manage your time effectively can help reduce stress by reducing the feeling of being overwhelmed. Make a to-do list, prioritize tasks, and delegate when possible.

- **Take breaks and relax:** Taking breaks and engaging in leisure activities, such as reading, taking a bath, or listening to music, can help reduce stress and improve overall well-being by providing a sense of balance.

- **Use hot or cold therapy:** Applying heat or cold to the affected area can help reduce pain and swelling.

- **Consider over-the-counter pain relievers:** Medications such as acetaminophen and ibuprofen can be effective in managing mild to moderate pain.

Remember, what works for one person may not work for another, so it's important to find what works best for you. Incorporating a combination of these strategies into your daily routine can help you reduce stress and improve your overall well-being.

Chapter 5

How to set realistic goals and maintain a positive outlook

Here are some tips for setting realistic goals and maintaining a positive outlook:

1. **Start small:** Break your larger goals into smaller, more manageable steps to avoid feeling overwhelmed.

2. **Be specific:** Make sure your goals are specific and measurable, so you can track your progress and see your achievements.

3. **Prioritize:** Choose the most important goals first and prioritize them, so you can focus your energy and resources on what is most important.

4. **Make a plan:** Write down a plan of action for each goal, including specific steps you need to take and deadlines.

5. **Stay positive:** Surround yourself with positive people, practice positive self-talk, and focus on the things that bring you joy and happiness.

6. **Celebrate your successes:** Recognize and celebrate your achievements, no matter how small

they may be, to keep your motivation and positive outlook high.

7. **Stay flexible:** Life is unpredictable, and your goals and plans may need to change along the way. Be open to new opportunities and be flexible in your approach to achieving your goals.

8. **Stay focused:** Avoid distractions and stay focused on your goals, but be sure to take breaks and give yourself time to recharge.

9. **Stay persistent:** Persistence and determination are key to achieving your goals. Stay focused and keep pushing forward, even when faced with challenges.

10. **Ask for help:** Don't be afraid to reach out for help or support when you need it. Surround yourself with people who believe in you and are there to help you reach your goals.

Strategies for staying active and engaged despite joint pain

Here are some strategies for staying active and engaged despite joint pain:

1. **Low-impact exercise:** Choose activities that put less strain on your joints, such as swimming, cycling, or water aerobics. These activities can help improve your flexibility and

strengthen your muscles without causing excessive pain.

2. **Gentle stretching:** Gentle stretching exercises can help improve joint mobility and reduce stiffness.

3. **Strength training:** Building up the muscles around your joints can help reduce the strain on those joints and improve your overall physical function.

4. **Aqua therapy:** Exercising in water can provide support and reduce the impact on your joints, making it a great option for those with joint pain.

5. **Tai Chi:** Tai Chi is a low-impact form of exercise that combines gentle movements with deep breathing and meditation. It has been shown to help reduce joint pain and improve physical function.

6. **Assistive devices:** Using assistive devices, such as a cane or knee brace, can help reduce the strain on your joints and make it easier for you to be active.

7. **Heat or cold therapy:** Applying heat or cold to your joints before and after physical activity can help reduce pain and swelling.

8. **Pacing yourself:** It's important to listen to your body and avoid pushing yourself too hard. Start with short, frequent sessions and gradually increase the duration and intensity of your physical activity over time.

9. **Adaptive sports:** There are many adaptive sports and recreation options available, such as seated volleyball or adaptive yoga, that can help you stay active and engaged while accommodating your joint pain.

10. **Stay mentally engaged:** In addition to physical activity, it's important to stay mentally engaged. Pursue hobbies, read, socialize with

friends, or take up a new hobby to stay mentally active and engaged.

Remember, it's important to work with your doctor to determine the best physical activity plan for you, taking into account the specific cause and severity of your joint pain.

Conclusion

The power of hope and healing is a concept that refers to the impact that a positive outlook and belief in the possibility of recovery can have on an individual's health and well-being. Research has shown that maintaining a sense of hope and optimism can have a profound effect on physical and mental health, and can play a key role in the healing process.

Hope and healing are closely connected, as hope provides the motivation and determination needed to overcome obstacles and make progress toward recovery. A positive outlook and belief in the possibility of healing can help individuals remain motivated and engaged in their treatment plan, even in the face of setbacks and challenges.

Additionally, hope and healing can also have a positive impact on an individual's emotional well-being. Feeling hopeful and optimistic can help reduce stress, anxiety, and depression, which can in turn improve physical health.

It's important to note that hope and healing are not a substitute for medical treatment, but rather a complementary approach to promoting health and well-being. A healthy dose of hope and positive thinking, combined with appropriate medical care, can provide individuals with the strength and resilience they need to overcome their challenges and achieve their goals.

The power of hope and healing is a powerful force that can have a significant impact on an individual's physical, mental, and emotional well-being. By maintaining a positive outlook and a belief in the possibility of recovery, individuals can enhance their ability to heal and live a fulfilling life.

"Rise Again: The Road to Recovery for Painful Joints" provides a comprehensive guide to managing joint pain and promoting healing. Through a detailed exploration of the causes and effects of joint pain, as well as an overview of medical and natural remedies, readers will gain a deeper understanding of their condition and the steps they can take to overcome it. Whether you are dealing with joint pain for the first time, or seeking new and innovative ways to manage your pain, this book offers practical advice and powerful strategies for regaining your mobility and improving your quality of life. With a combination of expert insights and personal experiences, "Rise Again" provides hope and inspiration for anyone looking to rise above joint pain and live a fulfilling, pain-free life.